SJOGREN SYNDROME DIET COOKBOOK FOR SENIORS

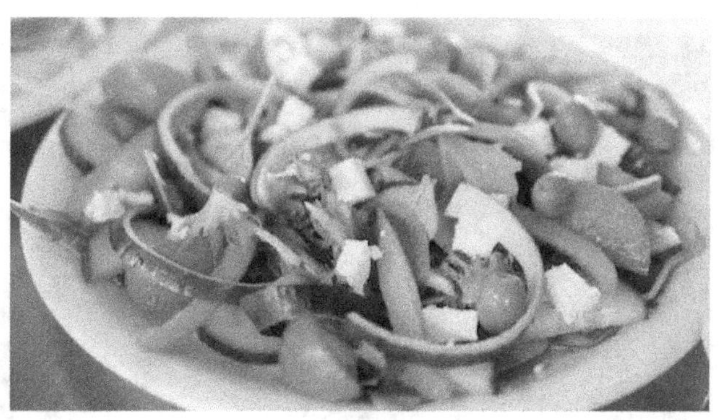

DR. JESSICA SMITH

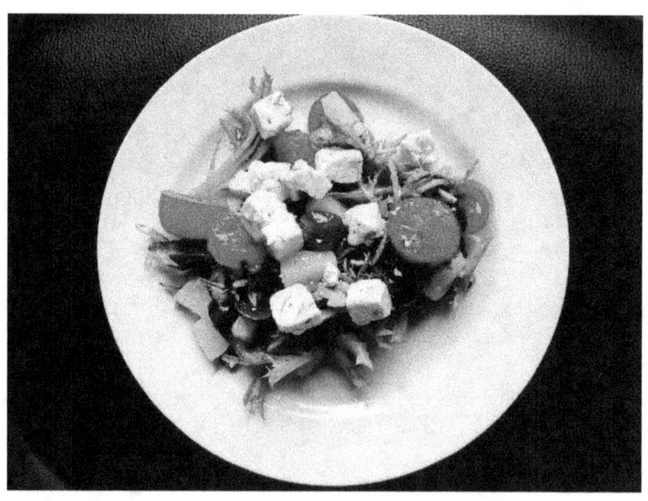

TABLE OF CONTENTS

CHAPTER ONE

How to Use this Cookbook

Understand the Basics:

Begin by familiarizing yourself with the basics of the Sjogren's Syndrome diet. Understand the principles of anti-inflammatory and nutrient-rich foods that can help alleviate symptoms associated with the condition.

Consult Your Healthcare Provider:

Before making significant changes to your diet, consult with your healthcare provider or a registered dietitian. They can provide personalized advice based on your specific health needs and conditions.

Explore the Recipe Categories:

The cookbook likely categorizes recipes based on meals (breakfast, lunch, dinner), snacks, and desserts. Take a moment to explore these categories and get an overview of the variety of recipes available.

Check for Dietary Restrictions: Pay attention to any dietary restrictions or modifications suggested in the cookbook. It might include information on gluten-free, dairy-free, or other specific dietary considerations that are relevant to managing Sjogren's Syndrome symptoms.

Create a Meal Plan:

Plan your meals for the week using the cookbook's recipes. Consider incorporating a variety of foods to ensure a well-balanced and nutrient-dense diet. A meal plan can make grocery shopping and preparation more straightforward.

Follow Serving Sizes and Portions:

Pay attention to serving sizes and portions recommended in the cookbook. Following appropriate portion control is crucial for maintaining a balanced diet and managing weight, which can be important for individuals with Sjogren's Syndrome.

Experiment with Substitutions:

If you have specific dietary preferences or restrictions, experiment with substitutions suggested in the cookbook. For example, explore alternative ingredients for allergens or ingredients that may trigger symptoms.

Keep a Food Diary:

Consider keeping a food diary to track how your body responds to different meals. Note any changes in symptoms, energy levels, or overall well-being. This information can be valuable during follow-up appointments with healthcare providers.

Stay Hydrated:

Given that Sjogren's Syndrome often leads to dryness, particularly in the mouth and eyes, stay mindful of your hydration. The cookbook may include tips on incorporating hydrating foods and beverages into your daily routine.

Understanding Sjogren Syndrome Diet

Understanding the Sjogren's Syndrome diet is paramount for individuals navigating this autoimmune condition, characterized by dryness in the eyes and mouth.

The diet is crafted to alleviate symptoms, reduce inflammation, and promote overall well-being. Key principles of the Sjogren's Syndrome diet involve incorporating anti-inflammatory foods and prioritizing nutrient-rich choices.

The cornerstone of this diet often revolves around hydration. Given the common symptom of dryness, staying well-hydrated is crucial.

The consumption of water-rich foods like fruits and vegetables, as well as maintaining a regular water intake, helps mitigate the effects of decreased saliva and tear production.

Moreover, the diet typically emphasizes omega-3 fatty acids found in fatty fish, flaxseeds, and walnuts.

These fatty acids possess anti-inflammatory properties, potentially aiding in managing the autoimmune response associated with Sjogren's Syndrome.

Additionally, antioxidant-rich foods, such as berries, dark leafy greens, and colorful vegetables, are encouraged to combat oxidative stress.

Dietary modifications may include reducing or eliminating potential triggers like gluten and dairy for those with sensitivities. It's crucial for individuals to work closely with healthcare professionals or dietitians to tailor the diet to their specific needs, considering factors like allergies, medications, and overall health.

Ultimately, the Sjogren's Syndrome diet serves as a tool to empower individuals in managing their symptoms, enhancing their quality of life, and promoting overall health.

Principles OF Sjogren Syndrome Diet

The principles of the Sjogren's Syndrome diet revolve around promoting anti-inflammatory properties, combating dryness, and supporting overall immune system health for individuals with this autoimmune condition. Key principles include:

Hydration is Key:

Adequate hydration is a fundamental principle to counteract the dryness associated with Sjogren's Syndrome. Water-rich foods, herbal teas, and regular water intake help address diminished saliva and tear production.

Anti-Inflammatory Foods:

The diet encourages the consumption of anti-inflammatory foods, such as fatty fish rich in omega-3 fatty acids (salmon, mackerel), flaxseeds, and walnuts. These elements may help alleviate inflammation associated with the autoimmune response.

Rich in Antioxidants:

Antioxidant-rich foods play a crucial role in the Sjogren's Syndrome diet. Berries, dark leafy greens, and vibrant vegetables are high in antioxidants, helping to neutralize oxidative stress and support immune function.

Omega-3 Fatty Acids:

Omega-3 fatty acids, found in certain fish, flaxseeds, and chia seeds, contribute to the diet's anti-inflammatory focus. These fats may help modulate the immune response and reduce inflammation in affected tissues.

Gluten and Dairy Considerations:

Some individuals with Sjogren's Syndrome may have sensitivities to gluten or dairy. The diet often considers these potential triggers, and modifications may involve reducing or eliminating them to manage symptoms effectively.

Balanced and Nutrient-Dense:

The overall diet encourages balance and nutrient density. This involves incorporating a variety of fruits, vegetables, whole grains, and lean proteins to ensure individuals receive a broad spectrum of essential vitamins and minerals.

Customization and Monitoring:

Recognizing the uniqueness of each individual's response to foods, the diet is highly customizable. Regular monitoring of symptoms and potential triggers is crucial to tailoring the diet to specific needs and ensuring its effectiveness over time.

Benefits of Sjogren Syndrome Diet

The benefits of the Sjogren's Syndrome diet extend beyond addressing the symptoms of dryness and discomfort associated with this autoimmune condition, offering a holistic approach to improved well-being.

Symptom Alleviation:

The foremost benefit lies in symptom alleviation. By focusing on anti-inflammatory and hydrating foods, individuals may experience relief from dry eyes and mouth, enhancing their overall comfort and quality of life.

Inflammation Reduction: The diet's emphasis on anti-inflammatory foods, such as omega-3 fatty acids and antioxidant-rich fruits and vegetables, may contribute to reducing overall inflammation in the body.

This can be particularly beneficial for managing the autoimmune response associated with Sjogren's Syndrome.

Improved Nutrient Intake:

The Sjogren's Syndrome diet promotes a nutrient-dense approach, ensuring individuals receive essential vitamins and minerals. This contributes to overall health and supports the immune system, which is often compromised in autoimmune conditions.

Customization for Individual Needs:

The diet's adaptable nature allows for customization based on individual sensitivities and preferences. Whether eliminating potential triggers like gluten and dairy or adjusting specific components, this flexibility ensures a personalized approach tailored to each person's unique requirements.

Enhanced Immune Function:

Antioxidants, omega-3 fatty acids, and other nutrients found in the recommended foods contribute to improved immune function.

Strengthening the immune system is vital for individuals with autoimmune conditions like Sjogren's Syndrome.

Positive Impact on Overall Health:

Beyond managing specific symptoms, the Sjogren's Syndrome diet can positively impact overall health. By fostering a balanced and nutritious diet, individuals may experience increased energy levels, better digestion, and a heightened sense of well-being.

Empowerment and Proactive Wellness:

Following the Sjogren's Syndrome diet empowers individuals to take an active role in managing their health. Making informed dietary choices and monitoring their body's responses instills a sense of control and proactive wellness in navigating the challenges of this autoimmune condition.

Tips for Sjogren Syndrome Diet

Adhering to the Sjogren's Syndrome diet can be a transformative journey for managing symptoms and promoting overall well-being.

Here are essential tips to navigate and optimize your experience with this specialized diet:

Stay Hydrated:

Prioritize hydration by consuming ample water and incorporating water-rich foods like cucumbers, watermelon, and oranges. This is crucial for mitigating the dryness associated with Sjogren's Syndrome.

Incorporate Omega-3 Fatty Acids:

Include sources of omega-3 fatty acids, such as fatty fish (salmon, trout), flaxseeds, and chia seeds, to combat inflammation and support overall immune health.

Embrace Antioxidant-Rich Foods: Prioritize colorful fruits and vegetables rich in antioxidants, like berries, spinach, and kale, to neutralize oxidative stress and bolster the immune system.

Consider Gluten and Dairy Sensitivities:

Assess whether gluten or dairy exacerbates symptoms and consider eliminating or reducing these components based on individual sensitivities.

Choose Nutrient-Dense Options:

Opt for nutrient-dense foods like whole grains, lean proteins, and legumes to ensure a well-rounded intake of essential vitamins and minerals.

Balance Macronutrients:

Strive for a balance of carbohydrates, proteins, and healthy fats in each meal to support sustained energy levels and overall nutrition.

Experiment with Cooking Methods:

Explore different cooking methods such as steaming, roasting, or grilling to enhance flavors and textures while retaining nutritional value.

Maintain Regular Monitoring: Keep a food diary to track how your body responds to different foods and identify potential triggers or patterns related to symptoms.

Collaborate with Healthcare Professionals:

Consult with your healthcare provider or a registered dietitian for personalized guidance and to address any concerns or questions about your dietary choices.

Be Mindful of Sugar Intake:

Monitor and limit added sugars, as excessive sugar consumption can contribute to inflammation and may impact overall health negatively.

Remember, the Sjogren's Syndrome diet is a tool for managing symptoms and promoting well-being, and its effectiveness may vary among individuals.

Guidelines for Sjogren Syndrome Diet

Following guidelines for the Sjogren's Syndrome diet can significantly impact symptom management and overall well-being. Here's a comprehensive set of guidelines to navigate this specialized diet effectively:

Prioritize Hydration:

Begin each day with water and incorporate hydrating foods like melons, cucumbers, and citrus fruits. Sip water throughout the day to combat dryness associated with Sjogren's Syndrome.

Include Omega-3 Fatty Acids: Regularly incorporate sources of omega-3 fatty acids, such as salmon, flaxseeds, and walnuts, to reduce inflammation and support immune function.

Emphasize Antioxidant-Rich Foods:

Consume a variety of colorful fruits and vegetables rich in antioxidants, like berries, spinach, and kale, to combat oxidative stress and bolster the immune system.

Limit Gluten and Dairy:

Evaluate individual tolerance to gluten and dairy, considering potential sensitivities. Some individuals with Sjogren's Syndrome find relief by reducing or eliminating these components.

Choose Nutrient-Dense Foods:

Opt for nutrient-dense options like whole grains, lean proteins, and legumes to ensure a well-rounded intake of essential vitamins and minerals.

Maintain Balanced Meals:

Aim for balanced meals that include a mix of carbohydrates, proteins, and healthy fats to support sustained energy levels and overall nutritional needs.

Experiment with Cooking Methods:

Explore various cooking methods such as steaming, roasting, or sautéing to enhance flavors while preserving the nutritional integrity of foods.

Monitor Sugar Intake:

Be mindful of added sugars in processed foods and beverages. Limiting sugar intake helps manage inflammation and supports overall health.

Keep a Food Diary: Track your dietary choices and note how your body responds to different foods. This can help identify patterns or triggers related to symptoms.

Consult Healthcare Professionals:

Regularly consult with healthcare providers or registered dietitians to receive personalized guidance, address concerns, and make informed decisions about your dietary choices.

Incorporate Hydrating Teas: Herbal teas, such as chamomile or peppermint, can contribute to hydration while providing soothing effects on the digestive system.

Mindful Eating Practices:

Practice mindful eating by savoring each bite, paying attention to hunger and fullness cues, and enjoying meals in a relaxed environment.

Adhering to these guidelines provides a framework for a well-balanced and nourishing Sjogren's Syndrome diet.

Causes of Sjogren Syndrome

Sjogren's Syndrome is an autoimmune disorder characterized by the immune system attacking the body's moisture-producing glands.

While the exact causes remain elusive, several factors are believed to contribute to the development of Sjogren's Syndrome:

Genetic Predisposition:

There appears to be a genetic component, as the risk of developing Sjogren's Syndrome is higher in individuals with a family history of autoimmune diseases.

Immune System Dysfunction: The disorder is primarily characterized by an abnormal immune response.

The immune system mistakenly identifies the body's own cells, particularly those in the glands producing saliva and tears, as foreign invaders, leading to chronic inflammation.

Hormonal Factors:

Hormonal influences, especially in women, have been implicated. The majority of individuals with Sjogren's Syndrome are women, suggesting a potential link to hormonal fluctuations.

Viral Infections: Exposure to certain viruses, such as Epstein-Barr virus (EBV) or cytomegalovirus (CMV), may trigger an immune response that contributes to the development of Sjogren's Syndrome.

Environmental Factors:

Environmental triggers, including exposure to certain toxins or infections, may play a role in initiating or exacerbating the autoimmune response.

Age:

Sjogren's Syndrome often manifests in individuals between the ages of 40 and 60, suggesting that age may be a contributing factor.

Understanding these potential causes provides a foundation for ongoing research aimed at unraveling the complexities of Sjogren's Syndrome.

While these factors are associated with the development of the condition, the interplay and precise mechanisms remain subjects of continued investigation in the scientific community.

Types of Sjogren Syndrome

Sjogren's Syndrome manifests in different forms, each varying in severity and associated symptoms. The two main types of Sjogren's Syndrome are primary and secondary:

Primary Sjogren's Syndrome:

In primary Sjogren's Syndrome, the condition occurs on its own, without being linked to any other autoimmune disorder. It primarily affects the exocrine glands responsible for producing moisture, leading to symptoms such as dry eyes, dry mouth, and dry skin.

Systemic manifestations can include joint pain, fatigue, and internal organ involvement.

Secondary Sjogren's Syndrome: Secondary Sjogren's Syndrome occurs alongside another autoimmune disorder, most commonly rheumatoid arthritis or systemic lupus erythematosus. Individuals with secondary

Sjogren's Syndrome often experience a more complex array of symptoms related to both Sjogren's and the coexisting autoimmune condition.

Within these two main types, Sjogren's Syndrome can be further categorized based on the extent of organ involvement and the severity of symptoms. Some individuals may primarily experience mild dryness, while others may face systemic complications affecting various organs.

Symptoms of Sjogren Syndrome

Sjogren's Syndrome manifests with a range of symptoms that primarily affect the body's moisture-producing glands. The hallmark symptoms include:

Dry Eyes:

Individuals with Sjogren's Syndrome often experience persistent dryness and irritation in the eyes, leading to discomfort, redness, and a gritty sensation.

Dry Mouth:

Reduced saliva production results in dryness of the mouth, contributing to difficulties in swallowing, speaking, and an increased risk of dental issues.

Dry Skin: The lack of moisture extends to the skin, causing dryness and potential skin problems.

Joint Pain and Swelling:

Sjogren's Syndrome can lead to joint pain, stiffness, and swelling, resembling symptoms seen in rheumatoid arthritis.

Fatigue:

Chronic fatigue is common and often stems from the body's immune response and inflammation.

Salivary Gland Enlargement:

Swelling of the salivary glands, particularly those located near the jaw, can occur.

Vaginal Dryness:

Women with Sjogren's Syndrome may experience dryness in the vaginal area, leading to discomfort during sexual activity.

Persistent Cough:

Dryness in the airways can result in a chronic cough.

Systemic Symptoms:

Some individuals may experience systemic symptoms such as fever, weight loss, and an overall feeling of malaise.

Organ Involvement:

In severe cases, Sjogren's Syndrome can affect internal organs, including the kidneys, lungs, and liver.

Symptoms can vary in intensity and may come and go over time. While Sjogren's Syndrome primarily affects the moisture-producing glands, it can also involve other systems, leading to a diverse range of manifestations.

Risk Factors of Sjogren Syndrome

Sjogren's Syndrome, like many autoimmune disorders, involves a complex interplay of genetic and environmental factors. Several risk factors contribute to the likelihood of developing this condition:

Gender: Sjogren's Syndrome predominantly affects women, with a significantly higher prevalence in females than males. The gender ratio is estimated to be around 9:1.

Age:

The risk of developing Sjogren's Syndrome increases with age, typically manifesting in individuals between the ages of 40 and 60. However, the condition can affect people of any age.

Genetic Predisposition:

There is a notable genetic component, as individuals with a family history of autoimmune diseases, including Sjogren's Syndrome, have a higher risk of developing the condition.

Other Autoimmune Disorders:

Having another autoimmune disorder, such as rheumatoid arthritis or systemic lupus erythematosus, increases the risk of developing Sjogren's Syndrome. This scenario is referred to as secondary Sjogren's Syndrome.

Viral Infections: Exposure to certain viruses, particularly Epstein-Barr virus (EBV), has been linked to an increased risk of developing Sjogren's Syndrome.

Viral infections may trigger an abnormal immune response that leads to the development of autoimmune disorders.

Environmental Factors: Environmental triggers, such as exposure to toxins or infections, may contribute to the initiation or exacerbation of Sjogren's Syndrome in genetically predisposed individuals.

Understanding these risk factors provides insights into the complex nature of Sjogren's Syndrome development.

It emphasizes the importance of comprehensive medical evaluation, particularly for individuals with a family history of autoimmune diseases or those experiencing symptoms associated with the condition.

CHAPTER TWO

Sjogren Syndrome Diet Breakfast Recipes for Seniors

1. Berry and Almond Smoothie Bowl

Ingredients:

- ➤ 1 cup mixed berries (blueberries, strawberries, raspberries)
- ➤ 1 banana
- ➤ 1/2 cup almond milk
- ➤ 2 tablespoons almond butter
- ➤ 1 tablespoon chia seeds
- ➤ 1 tablespoon honey (optional)

Instructions:

- ➤ Blend berries, banana, almond milk, almond butter, and chia seeds until smooth.
- ➤ Pour into a bowl and top with additional berries and a drizzle of honey.

Health Benefits:

> ➤ Rich in antioxidants, omega-3 fatty acids, and vitamins.
> ➤ Supports hydration and immune function.

Preparation Time: 10 minutes

2. Quinoa Breakfast Porridge

Ingredients:

> ➤ 1/2 cup quinoa, rinsed
> ➤ 1 cup almond milk
> ➤ 1/2 teaspoon cinnamon
> ➤ 1/4 cup chopped nuts (almonds, walnuts)
> ➤ 1 tablespoon maple syrup
> ➤ Fresh fruit for topping

Instructions:

> ➤ Cook quinoa in almond milk with cinnamon until fluffy.
> ➤ Stir in nuts and maple syrup.
> ➤ Top with fresh fruit.
> ➤ Health Benefits: Quinoa provides protein, fiber, and essential nutrients. Nuts offer healthy fats.

Preparation Time: 15 minutes

3. Avocado and Tomato Toast

Ingredients:

- ➢ 2 slices whole grain bread
- ➢ 1 ripe avocado
- ➢ 1 medium tomato, sliced
- ➢ Fresh basil leaves
- ➢ Salt and pepper to taste

Instructions:

- ➢ Toast bread slices.
- ➢ Mash avocado and spread over the toast.
- ➢ Top with tomato slices, basil, salt, and pepper.

Health Benefits:

- ➢ Avocado provides healthy fats, while tomatoes offer antioxidants.

Preparation Time: 10 minutes

4. Chia Seed Pudding with Berries

Ingredients:

- 3 tablespoons chia seeds
- 1 cup almond milk
- 1/2 teaspoon vanilla extract
- Mixed berries for topping

Instructions:

- Mix chia seeds, almond milk, and vanilla extract in a jar.
- Refrigerate overnight.
- Top with mixed berries before serving.

Health Benefits:

- Chia seeds are rich in omega-3s and fiber.

Preparation Time: 5 minutes (plus overnight chilling)

5. Spinach and Feta Omelette

Ingredients:

- 2 eggs
- Handful of fresh spinach

- ➢ 2 tablespoons crumbled feta cheese

- ➢ Salt and pepper to taste

- ➢ Olive oil for cooking

Instructions:

- ➢ Whisk eggs and pour into a heated skillet.

- ➢ Add spinach and feta. Cook until set.

- ➢ Fold and serve.

Health Benefits:

- ➢ Spinach provides iron, while eggs offer protein.

Preparation Time: 10 minutes

6. Greek Yogurt Parfait

Ingredients:

- ➢ 1 cup Greek yogurt

- ➢ Granola

- ➢ Mixed berries

- ➢ Honey for drizzling

Instructions:

- ➢ Layer Greek yogurt, granola, and berries in a glass.

- ➢ Repeat layers.
- ➢ Drizzle with honey before serving.

Health Benefits:

- ➢ Greek yogurt provides probiotics, and berries offer antioxidants.

Preparation Time: 5 minutes

7. Sweet Potato Breakfast Hash

Ingredients:

- ➢ 1 sweet potato, diced
- ➢ 1/2 red bell pepper, diced
- ➢ 1/4 red onion, diced
- ➢ 1 tablespoon olive oil
- ➢ 1/2 teaspoon smoked paprika
- ➢ Salt and pepper to taste

Instructions:

- ➢ Sauté sweet potato, bell pepper, and onion in olive oil until tender.
- ➢ Season with smoked paprika, salt, and pepper.

Health Benefits:

> Sweet potatoes provide vitamins, and bell peppers offer antioxidants.

Preparation Time: 15 minutes

8. Banana Nut Overnight Oats

Ingredients:

> 1/2 cup rolled oats
> 1/2 cup almond milk
> 1 ripe banana, mashed
> 2 tablespoons chopped nuts (walnuts, almonds)
> 1/2 teaspoon cinnamon

Instructions:

> Mix oats, almond milk, mashed banana, nuts, and cinnamon in a jar.
> Refrigerate overnight.

Health Benefits:

> Oats offer fiber, and bananas provide potassium.

Preparation Time: 5 minutes (plus overnight chilling)

9. Cottage Cheese and Pineapple Bowl

Ingredients:

- 1 cup low-fat cottage cheese
- 1 cup fresh pineapple chunks
- 1 tablespoon shredded coconut

Instructions:

- Combine cottage cheese and pineapple in a bowl.
- Top with shredded coconut.

Health Benefits:

- Cottage cheese offers protein, and pineapple provides vitamin C.

Preparation Time: 5 minutes

10. Almond Butter and Banana Wrap

Ingredients:

- 1 whole grain tortilla
- 2 tablespoons almond butter
- 1 banana, sliced
- Drizzle of honey

Instructions:

- ➢ Spread almond butter on the tortilla.
- ➢ Add banana slices and drizzle with honey.
- ➢ Roll into a wrap.
- ➢ Health Benefits: Almond butter provides healthy fats, and bananas offer potassium.

Preparation Time: 5 minutes

Sjogren Syndrome Diet Lunch Recipes for Seniors

1. Quinoa Salad with Roasted Vegetables

Ingredients:

- ➢ 1 cup cooked quinoa
- ➢ Mixed roasted vegetables (bell peppers, zucchini, cherry tomatoes)
- ➢ Feta cheese
- ➢ Fresh basil
- ➢ Olive oil, balsamic vinegar
- ➢ Salt and pepper to taste

Instructions:

> ➢ Toss cooked quinoa with roasted vegetables.
> ➢ Add feta cheese and fresh basil.
> ➢ Dress with olive oil, balsamic vinegar, salt, and pepper.

Health Benefits:

> ➢ Quinoa offers protein, and vegetables provide vitamins and antioxidants.

Preparation Time: 20 minutes

2. Salmon and Avocado Wrap

Ingredients:

> ➢ Grilled salmon fillet
> ➢ Whole grain wrap
> ➢ Sliced avocado
> ➢ Spinach leaves
> ➢ Greek yogurt sauce
> ➢ Lemon juice

Instructions:

> Place grilled salmon, avocado, and spinach on a whole grain wrap.
> Drizzle with Greek yogurt sauce and lemon juice.
> Roll into a wrap.

Health Benefits:

> Salmon provides omega-3 fatty acids, and avocados offer healthy fats.

Preparation Time: 15 minutes

3. Lentil and Vegetable Soup

Ingredients:

> 1 cup dried lentils
> Mixed vegetables (carrots, celery, onions)
> Vegetable broth
> Garlic, thyme, cumin
> Fresh parsley for garnish

Instructions:

> Cook lentils with mixed vegetables in vegetable broth.

➢ Season with garlic, thyme, and cumin.

➢ Garnish with fresh parsley.

Health Benefits:

➢ Lentils provide protein, and vegetables offer vitamins.

Preparation Time: 30 minutes

4. Turkey and Quinoa Stuffed Peppers

Ingredients:

➢ Bell peppers, halved

➢ Ground turkey

➢ Cooked quinoa

➢ Tomato sauce

➢ Italian seasoning

➢ Mozzarella cheese

Instructions:

➢ Mix ground turkey with cooked quinoa, tomato sauce, and Italian seasoning.

➢ Stuff bell peppers with the mixture.

➢ Top with mozzarella cheese and bake until bubbly.

Health Benefits:

Turkey is a lean protein, and quinoa provides essential nutrients.

Preparation Time: 40 minutes

5. Spinach and Chickpea Salad

Ingredients:

- ➤ Fresh spinach leaves
- ➤ Chickpeas (canned, drained)
- ➤ Cherry tomatoes, halved
- ➤ Cucumber, sliced
- ➤ Red onion, thinly sliced
- ➤ Olive oil, lemon juice, Dijon mustard

Instructions:

- ➤ Combine spinach, chickpeas, tomatoes, cucumber, and red onion in a bowl.
- ➤ Dress with a mixture of olive oil, lemon juice, and Dijon mustard.

Health Benefits:

> ➤ Spinach offers iron, and chickpeas provide protein and fiber.

Preparation Time: 15 minutes

6. Grilled Chicken and Quinoa Bowl

Ingredients:

> ➤ Grilled chicken breast
> ➤ Quinoa
> ➤ Steamed broccoli
> ➤ Avocado slices
> ➤ Lemon-tahini dressing

Instructions:

> ➤ Arrange grilled chicken, quinoa, steamed broccoli, and avocado in a bowl.
> ➤ Drizzle with lemon-tahini dressing.

Health Benefits:

> ➤ Chicken offers protein, and quinoa provides a complete source of protein.

Preparation Time: 25 minutes

7. Eggplant and Tomato Stew

Ingredients:

- Eggplant, diced
- Tomatoes, diced
- Garlic, onion, bell peppers
- Vegetable broth
- Paprika, cumin, coriander
- Fresh cilantro for garnish

Instructions:

- Sauté eggplant, tomatoes, garlic, onion, and bell peppers in a pot.
- Add vegetable broth and season with paprika, cumin, and coriander.
- Garnish with fresh cilantro.

Health Benefits:

- Eggplant offers antioxidants, and tomatoes provide vitamins.

Preparation Time: 30 minutes

8. Shrimp and Quinoa Stir-Fry

Ingredients:

- Shrimp, peeled and deveined
- Quinoa
- Mixed vegetables (broccoli, bell peppers, snap peas)
- Soy sauce, ginger, garlic
- Sesame oil

Instructions:

- Stir-fry shrimp and mixed vegetables in sesame oil with ginger and garlic.
- Add cooked quinoa and soy sauce.

Health Benefits:

- Shrimp offers protein, and quinoa provides essential nutrients.

Preparation Time: 20 minutes

9. Mediterranean Chickpea Salad

Ingredients:

- Canned chickpeas, drained

➤ Cherry tomatoes, halved

➤ Cucumber, diced

➤ Kalamata olives, sliced

➤ Feta cheese

➤ Olive oil, lemon juice, oregano

Instructions:

➤ Mix chickpeas, tomatoes, cucumber, olives, and feta in a bowl.

➤ Dress with olive oil, lemon juice, and oregano.

Health Benefits:

➤ Chickpeas offer protein, and vegetables provide vitamins and antioxidants.

Preparation Time: 15 minutes

10. Butternut Squash and Kale Salad

Ingredients:

➤ Roasted butternut squash cubes

➤ Kale, chopped

➤ Pomegranate seeds

➤ Goat cheese

- ➢ Balsamic vinaigrette

Instructions:

- ➢ Combine roasted butternut squash, kale, pomegranate seeds, and goat cheese in a bowl.
- ➢ Drizzle with balsamic vinaigrette.

Health Benefits:

- ➢ Butternut squash provides vitamins, and kale offers iron.

Preparation Time: 25 minutes

Sjogren Syndrome Diet Dinner Recipes for Seniors

1. Baked Lemon Garlic Salmon

Ingredients:

- ➢ Salmon fillets
- ➢ Lemon slices
- ➢ Minced garlic
- ➢ Fresh dill
- ➢ Olive oil

> Salt and pepper to taste

Instructions:

> Place salmon fillets on a baking sheet.

> Top with lemon slices, minced garlic, and fresh dill.

> Drizzle with olive oil, season with salt and pepper.

> Bake until salmon is cooked through.

Health Benefits:

> Salmon provides omega-3 fatty acids, and garlic offers anti-inflammatory properties.

Preparation Time: 20 minutes

2. Quinoa and Vegetable Stuffed Bell Peppers

Ingredients:

> Bell peppers, halved

> Cooked quinoa

> Mixed vegetables (zucchini, cherry tomatoes, corn)

> Tomato sauce

> Italian herbs

> Mozzarella cheese

Instructions:

- ➤ Mix cooked quinoa with mixed vegetables, tomato sauce, and Italian herbs.
- ➤ Stuff bell peppers with the quinoa mixture.
- ➤ Top with mozzarella cheese and bake until cheese melts.

Health Benefits:

- ➤ Quinoa offers protein, and vegetables provide vitamins.

Preparation Time: 30 minutes

3. Chicken and Vegetable Stir-Fry

Ingredients:

- ➤ Chicken breast, sliced
- ➤ Broccoli florets
- ➤ Bell peppers, sliced
- ➤ Snap peas
- ➤ Soy sauce, ginger, garlic
- ➤ Brown rice

Instructions:

> Stir-fry sliced chicken with broccoli, bell peppers, and snap peas.
> Add soy sauce, ginger, and garlic.
> Serve over cooked brown rice.

Health Benefits:

> Chicken provides protein, and vegetables offer vitamins.

Preparation Time: 25 minutes

4. Lentil and Sweet Potato Curry

Ingredients:

> Red lentils
> Sweet potatoes, diced
> Coconut milk
> Curry spices (turmeric, cumin, coriander)
> Spinach leaves
> Fresh cilantro for garnish

Instructions:

> Cook red lentils and sweet potatoes in coconut milk with curry spices.
> Add spinach leaves and cook until wilted.
> Garnish with fresh cilantro.

Health Benefits:

> Lentils provide protein, and sweet potatoes offer vitamins.

Preparation Time: 35 minutes

5. Turkey and Vegetable Skewers

Ingredients:

> Ground turkey
> Bell peppers, onions, cherry tomatoes
> Olive oil, lemon juice
> Italian herbs
> Quinoa

Instructions:

> Mix ground turkey with Italian herbs.

- ➢ Form into skewers with bell peppers, onions, and cherry tomatoes.
- ➢ Grill until turkey is cooked through.
- ➢ Serve over cooked quinoa, drizzle with olive oil and lemon juice.

Health Benefits:

- ➢ Turkey provides lean protein, and vegetables offer vitamins.

Preparation Time: 30 minutes

6. Mediterranean Grilled Eggplant Salad

Ingredients:

- ➢ Sliced eggplant
- ➢ Cherry tomatoes, halved
- ➢ Cucumber, diced
- ➢ Kalamata olives, sliced
- ➢ Feta cheese
- ➢ Olive oil, lemon juice, oregano

Instructions:

- ➢ Grill sliced eggplant until tender.

➢ Combine with cherry tomatoes, cucumber, olives, and feta.

➢ Dress with olive oil, lemon juice, and oregano.

Health Benefits:

➢ Eggplant offers antioxidants, and olives provide healthy fats.

Preparation Time: 25 minutes

7. Shrimp and Vegetable Zoodle Stir-Fry

Ingredients:

➢ Shrimp, peeled and deveined

➢ Zucchini noodles (zoodles)

➢ Carrots, julienned

➢ Snow peas

➢ Sesame oil, soy sauce, ginger

➢ Sesame seeds for garnish

Instructions:

➢ Stir-fry shrimp with zucchini noodles, julienned carrots, and snow peas.

➢ Add sesame oil, soy sauce, and ginger.

> Garnish with sesame seeds.

Health Benefits:

> Shrimp provides protein, and zucchini offers
> vitamins.

Preparation Time: 20 minutes

8. Tomato Basil Chickpea Pasta

Ingredients:

> Chickpea pasta
> Cherry tomatoes, halved
> Fresh basil leaves
> Garlic, olive oil, red pepper flakes
> Parmesan cheese (optional)

Instructions:

> Cook chickpea pasta according to package
> instructions.
> Sauté cherry tomatoes, garlic, and red pepper flakes
> in olive oil.
> Toss with cooked pasta and fresh basil.
> Optional: sprinkle with Parmesan cheese.

Health Benefits:

> ➢ Chickpea pasta provides protein, and tomatoes offer antioxidants.

Preparation Time: 15 minutes

9. Spinach and Feta Stuffed Chicken Breast

Ingredients:

> ➢ Chicken breasts
> ➢ Fresh spinach leaves
> ➢ Feta cheese
> ➢ Garlic, lemon zest, olive oil
> ➢ Paprika, salt, and pepper

Instructions:

> ➢ Butterfly chicken breasts and stuff with spinach and feta.
> ➢ Season with garlic, lemon zest, paprika, salt, and pepper.
> ➢ Bake until chicken is cooked through.

Health Benefits:

> ➢ Chicken offers protein, and spinach provides iron.

Preparation Time: 30 minutes

10. Cauliflower Rice Stir-Fry with Tofu

Ingredients:

- ➢ Cauliflower rice
- ➢ Extra-firm tofu, cubed
- ➢ Mixed vegetables (broccoli, carrots, peas)
- ➢ Soy sauce, ginger, garlic
- ➢ Green onions for garnish

Instructions:

- ➢ Stir-fry tofu and mixed vegetables in a pan with soy sauce, ginger, and garlic.
- ➢ Add cauliflower rice and cook until heated through.
- ➢ Garnish with green onions.

Health Benefits:

- ➢ Tofu provides protein, and cauliflower offers a low-carb alternative.

Preparation Time: 25 minutes

1. Hummus and Veggie Sticks

Ingredients:

- ➤ Hummus
- ➤ Carrot sticks, cucumber slices, bell pepper strips
- ➤ Cherry tomatoes

Instructions:

- ➤ Arrange veggie sticks around a bowl of hummus.
- ➤ Dip and enjoy!

Health Benefits:

- ➤ Hummus provides protein, and veggies offer vitamins and antioxidants.

Preparation Time: 10 minutes

2. Greek Yogurt Parfait with Berries

Ingredients:

- ➤ Greek yogurt

- ➢ Granola
- ➢ Mixed berries (blueberries, strawberries)
- ➢ Honey

Instructions:

- ➢ Layer Greek yogurt, granola, and berries in a glass.
- ➢ Drizzle with honey.

Health Benefits:

- ➢ Greek yogurt offers probiotics, and berries provide antioxidants.

Preparation Time: 5 minutes

3. Almond Butter and Banana Rice Cakes

Ingredients:

- ➢ Rice cakes
- ➢ Almond butter
- ➢ Sliced banana
- ➢ Chia seeds

Instructions:

- ➢ Spread almond butter on rice cakes.

➤ Top with sliced banana and sprinkle with chia seeds.

Health Benefits:

➤ Almond butter provides healthy fats, and bananas offer potassium.

Preparation Time: 5 minutes

4. Avocado and Tomato Salsa

Ingredients:

➤ Avocado, diced

➤ Tomatoes, diced

➤ Red onion, finely chopped

➤ Cilantro, chopped

➤ Lime juice

➤ Whole grain tortilla chips

Instructions:

➤ Mix avocado, tomatoes, red onion, and cilantro.

➤ Add lime juice and serve with whole grain tortilla chips.

Health Benefits: Avocado provides healthy fats, and tomatoes offer vitamins.

Preparation Time: 10 minutes

5. Trail Mix with Nuts and Dried Fruits

Ingredients:

- Almonds, walnuts, pistachios
- Dried cranberries, apricots, raisins
- Dark chocolate chips

Instructions:

- Mix nuts, dried fruits, and dark chocolate chips in a bowl.
- Portion into small snack bags.

Health Benefits:

- Nuts provide healthy fats, and dried fruits offer natural sweetness.

Preparation Time: 5 minutes

6. Cottage Cheese and Pineapple Bowl

Ingredients:

- Low-fat cottage cheese
- Fresh pineapple chunks

➤ Shredded coconut

Instructions:

➤ Combine cottage cheese and pineapple in a bowl.

➤ Top with shredded coconut.

Health Benefits:

➤ Cottage cheese offers protein, and pineapple provides vitamin C.

Preparation Time: 5 minutes

7. Baked Sweet Potato Chips

Ingredients:

➤ Sweet potatoes, thinly sliced

➤ Olive oil

➤ Paprika, garlic powder

➤ Sea salt

Instructions:

➤ Toss sweet potato slices in olive oil and season with paprika and garlic powder.

➤ Bake until crispy.

> Sprinkle with sea salt before serving.

Health Benefits:

> Sweet potatoes provide vitamins, and olive oil offers healthy fats.

Preparation Time: 25 minutes

8. Edamame and Sea Salt

Ingredients:

> Edamame beans (frozen, thawed)

> Sea salt

Instructions:

> Steam or boil edamame beans until tender.

> Sprinkle with sea salt.

Health Benefits:

> Edamame provides protein and fiber.

Preparation Time: 10 minutes

9. Cucumber and Tzatziki Bites

Ingredients:

- ➤ Cucumber slices
- ➤ Tzatziki sauce
- ➤ Dill for garnish

Instructions:

- ➤ Top cucumber slices with a dollop of tzatziki sauce.
- ➤ Garnish with dill.

Health Benefits:

- ➤ Cucumbers offer hydration, and tzatziki provides probiotics.

Preparation Time: 10 minutes

10. Apple and Almond Butter Sandwiches

Ingredients:

- ➤ Apple slices
- ➤ Almond butter
- ➤ Granola

Instructions:

- ➤ Spread almond butter on apple slices.
- ➤ Sprinkle with granola and sandwich together.

Health Benefits:

- ➤ Apples provide fiber, and almond butter offers healthy fats.

CONCLUSION

The Sjogren's Syndrome Diet Cookbook is more than just a collection of recipes; it's a guide to embracing a lifestyle that supports overall well-being for individuals navigating the challenges of this autoimmune condition.

Our culinary journey has been a celebration of flavor, nourishment, and thoughtful choices that align with the principles of managing Sjogren's Syndrome.

As we've explored a myriad of breakfasts, lunches, dinners, and snacks, the emphasis has always been on anti-inflammatory ingredients, hydration, and nutrient-rich options.

From vibrant salads to wholesome soups, each recipe is carefully crafted to contribute to a diet that may help alleviate symptoms, promote immune health, and enhance overall vitality.

This cookbook extends beyond the kitchen, encouraging mindfulness about what we put into our bodies. It stands as a testament to the empowering notion that food can be both medicine and a source of joy.

By making informed choices and savoring every bite, individuals with Sjogren's Syndrome can cultivate a positive relationship with their diets, paving the way for a healthier and more enjoyable life.

Let this cookbook be a constant companion, providing inspiration and practical solutions for those embracing a Sjogren's-friendly lifestyle.

May these recipes not only nourish the body but also nourish the spirit, fostering a sense of resilience, balance, and satisfaction. Here's to savoring every delicious moment on the path to well-being.